Ketogenic Slow Cooker Cookbook For Beginners

Easy Cookbook With Quick & Delicious Recipes to Stay Healthy and Enjoy Taste Slow Cooker Dishes to Lose Weight Loss

Jasmine Reyes

Disclaimer Notice:

Please note the information contained within this document is for educational and entertainment purposes only. All effort has been executed to present accurate, up to date, and reliable, complete information. No warranties of any kind are declared or implied. Readers acknowledge that the author is not engaging in the rendering of legal, financial, medical or professional advice. The content within this book has been derived from various sources. Please consult a licensed professional before attempting any techniques outlined in this book.

By reading this document, the reader agrees that under no circumstances is the author responsible for any losses, direct or indirect, which are incurred as a result of the use of information contained within this document, including, but not limited to, errors, omissions, or inaccuracies.

Table of Content

Introduction

Thank you for purchasing **Ketogenic Slow Cooker Cookbook For Beginners: Easy Cookbook With Quick & Delicious Recipes to Stay Healthy and Enjoy Taste Slow Cooker Dishes to Lose Weight Loss**

Having a slow stove is an effortless, fast and more flexible method of cooking in any home. It doesn't require any cooking skills; it saves your time because the slow cooker does all the work time for you, it's really safe and it can also be used in any place like a hotel room or even a student dorm because it has a kettle like shape, making it more portable than a stove. So, in the following guides, we will discuss some of the basic ways that are useful to ensure that you get the best out of your slow stove.

What it is.

The slow cooker appeared in 1970 and was marketed as a bean pot. But as it was modified, people started using it to reheat food and keep it warm for extended periods. And look how far we've come: people are cooking delicious, healthy meals with it. It's a perfect little kitchen appliance that consists of a glass lid, porcelain or ceramic pot (it's inside the heating unit) and, of course, a heating element. The modern Slow Cooker can be oval or round in shape and various sizes from small to large. All Slow Cookers have two settings: LOW (corresponds to a temperature of 200°F mostly) and HIGH (up to 300°F). The WARM selection found among most slow cooker options these days allows you to keep prepared dishes warm for a long time. Some slow cooker models have a timer that will allow you to control the cooking time if you are busy.

Breakfast Recipes

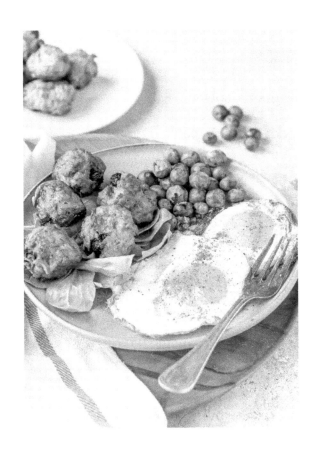

Bacon & Cheese Frittata

Preparation Time: 15 minutes

Cooking time: 2 hours 30 minutes Servings: 8

Ingredients:

- 1/2 lb bacon

- 2 tablespoons butter

- 8 oz fresh spinach, packed down

- 10 eggs

- 1/2 cup heavy whipping cream

- 1/2 cup shredded cheese

- Salt and pepper

Directions:

1. Butter or grease the inside of your slow-cooker.

2. Loosely chop the spinach.

3. Cut bacon into half-inch pieces.

4. Beat the eggs with the spices, cream, cheese, and chopped spinach. Then everything will be blended smoothly. Line the bottom of the slow cooker with the bacon.

5. Pour the egg mixture over the bacon.

6. Cover the crock pot and adjust the temperature to high

7. Cook for 2 hours. Serve hot.

Nutrition: calories 392, fat 34, carbs 4, protein 19

Delight Breakfast Meatloaf

Preparation Time: 10 minutes   Cooking time: 3 hours 10 minutes   Servings: 8

Ingredients:

- 2 lb ground pork

- 2 eggs

- 2 tbsp paprika

- 2 tbsp fresh sage

- 1 tbsp olive oil

- 1 diced onion

- 3 garlic cloves

- 1/4 cup of almond flour

Directions:

1. Saute vegetables in the slow cooker in the olive oil until brown.

2. Mix the pork, eggs, sage, paprika, and almond flour, thoroughly.

3. Add the cooked onions and garlic.

4. Shape the meat mixture into the shape of a loaf.

5.   Put the loaf in the slow cooker, cover with the lid and cook for three hours on low heat.

6.   Serve in slices immediately or save to serve at breakfast later.

Nutrition: calories 406, fat 26, carbs 5, protein 32

Low-Carb Hash Brown Breakfast Casserole

Preparation Time: 10 minutes

Cooking time: 6 hours on low

Servings: 6

Ingredients:

• 1 tablespoon unsalted butter, Ghee (here), or extra-virgin olive oil

• 12 large eggs

• ½ cup heavy (whipping) cream

• ½ teaspoon ground mustard

• 1 head cauliflower, shredded or minced

• 1 onion, diced

• 10 ounces cooked breakfast sausage links, sliced

• 2 cups shredded Cheddar cheese, divided

Directions:

1. Generously coat the inside of the slow cooker insert with the butter.

2.   In a large bowl, beat the eggs, then whisk in heavy cream, 1 teaspoon of salt, ½ teaspoon of pepper, and the ground mustard.

3.   Spread about one-third of the cauliflower in an even layer in the bottom of the cooker.

4.   Layer one-third of the onions over the cauliflower, then one-third of the sausage, and top with ½ cup of Cheddar cheese. Season with salt and pepper. Repeat twice more with the remaining ingredients. You should have ½ cup of Cheddar cheese left.

5.   Pour the egg mixture evenly over the layered ingredients, then sprinkle the remaining ½ cup Cheddar cheese on top. Cover and cook for 6 hours on low. Serve hot.

Nutrition: calories 523, fat 18, carbs 7, protein 3

Asparagus Smoked Salmon

Preparation Time: 15 minutes

Cooking time: 5 hours

Servings: 6

Ingredients:

- 1 tablespoon extra-virgin olive oil

- 6 large eggs

- 1 cup heavy (whipping) cream

- 2 teaspoons chopped fresh dill, plus additional for garnish

- ½ teaspoon kosher salt

- ¼ teaspoon freshly ground black pepper

- 1½ cups shredded Havarti or Monterey Jack cheese

- 12 ounces asparagus, trimmed and sliced

- 6 ounces smoked salmon, flaked

- Generously coat the inside of the slow cooker insert with the olive oil.

- In a large bowl, beat the eggs, then whisk in the heavy cream, dill, salt, and pepper.

- Stir in the cheese and asparagus.

Directions:

1.   Gently fold in the salmon and then pour the mixture
into the prepared insert.

2.   Cover and cook for 6 hours on low or 3 hours on high.

3.   Serve warm, garnished with additional fresh dill.

Nutrition: calories 388, fat 19, carbs 10, protein 21

Lunch Recipes

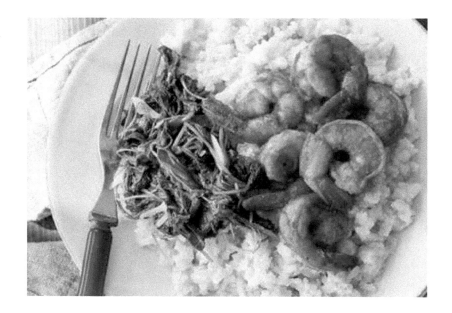

Parmesan Potato with Dill

Preparation time: 17 minutes

Cooking time: 4 hours

Servings: 5

Ingredients:

- 1-pound small potato

- ½ cup fresh dill

- 7 oz. Parmesan

- 1 teaspoon rosemary

- 1 teaspoon thyme

- 1 cup water

- ¼ teaspoon chili flakes

- 3 tablespoon cream

- 1 teaspoon salt

Directions:

1. Peel the potatoes and put them in the slow cooker.

2. Add water, salt, thyme, rosemary, and chili flakes.

3. Close the slow cooker lid and cook the potato for 2 hours on HIGH.

4.   Meanwhile, shred Parmesan cheese and chop the fresh dill. When the time is done, sprinkle the potato with the cream and fresh dill. Stir it carefully.

5.   Add shredded Parmesan cheese and close the slow cooker lid. Cook the potato on HIGH for 2 hours more.

6.   Then open the slow cooker lid and do not stir the potato anymore. Gently transfer the dish to the serving plates. Enjoy!

Nutrition:

Calories 235,

Fat 3.9,

Fiber 2,

Carbs 32.26,

Protein 1

Light Taco Soup

Preparation time: 24 minutes

Cooking time: 7 hours

Servings: 5

Ingredients:

- 7 oz. ground chicken

- ½ teaspoon sesame oil

- 3 cup vegetable stock

- 3 oz. yellow onion

- 1 cup tomato, canned

- 3 tomatoes

- 5 oz. corn kernels

- 1 jalapeno pepper, sliced

- ½ cup white beans, drained

- 3 tablespoon taco seasoning

- ¼ teaspoon salt

- 3 oz. black olives, sliced

- 5 corn tortillas, for serving

Directions:

1.   Peel the onion and dice it. Chop the fresh and canned tomatoes.

2.   Place the ground chicken, sesame oil, vegetable stock, diced onion, chopped tomatoes, sliced black olives, sliced jalapeno pepper, and corn in the slow cooker.

3.   Add the white beans, taco seasoning, and salt.

4.   Stir the soup mixture gently and close the slow cooker lid.

5.   Cook the soup for 7 hours on LOW. Meanwhile, cut the corn tortillas into the strips and bake them in the preheated to 365 F oven for 10 minutes.

6.   When the soup is cooked, ladle it into the serving bowls and sprinkle with the baked corn tortilla strips. Enjoy!

Nutrition:

Calories 328,

Fat 9.6,

Fiber 10,

Carbs 45.19,

Protein 18

Onion Lunch Muffins

Preparation time: 15 minutes

Cooking time: 8 hours

Servings: 7

Ingredients:

- 1 egg
- 5 tablespoons butter, melted
- 1 cup flour
- ½ cup milk
- 1 teaspoon baking soda
- 1 cup onion, chopped
- 1 teaspoon cilantro
- ½ teaspoon sage
- 1 teaspoon apple cider vinegar
- 2 cup water
- 1 tablespoon chives
- 1 teaspoon olive oil

Directions:

1. Beat the egg in the bowl and add melted butter.

2.   Add the flour, baking soda, chopped onion, milk, sage, apple cider vinegar, cilantro, and chives. Knead into a dough.

3.   After this, spray a muffin form with the olive oil inside. Fill the ½ part of every muffin form and place them in the glass jars.

4.   After this, pour water in the slow cooker vessel.

5.   Place the glass jars with muffins in the slow cooker and close the lid.

6.   Cook the muffins for 8 hours on LOW.

7.   Check if the muffins are cooked with the help of the toothpick and remove them from the slow cooker. Enjoy the dish warm!

Nutrition:

Calories 180,

Fat 11,

Fiber 1,

Carbs 16.28,

Protein 4

Lemon Orzo

Preparation time: 20 minutes

Cooking time: 2 hours 30 minutes

Servings: 5

Ingredients:

- 4 oz. shallot

- 7 oz. orzo

- 2 cup chicken stock

- 1 teaspoon paprika

- 1 teaspoon ground black pepper

- 1 teaspoon salt

- 1 lemon

- ¼ cup cream

- 2 yellow sweet pepper

- 1 cup baby spinach

Directions:

1. Chop the shallot and place it in the slow cooker.

2. Add the chicken stock and paprika. Sprinkle the mixture with the ground black pepper and salt. Stir it gently and cook on HIGH for 30 minutes.

3.   Meanwhile, grate the zest from the lemon and squeeze the juice. Add the lemon zest and juice in the slow cooker and stir it. After this, chop the baby spinach.

4.   Add it into the slow cooker. Remove the seeds from the yellow sweet peppers and chop into tiny pieces. Add the chopped peppers to the slow cooker.

5.   Add orzo and heavy cream. Stir the mass carefully and close the slow cooker lid. Cook the dish for 2 hours on LOW. Mixthe dish gently. Enjoy!

Nutrition:

Calories 152,

Fat 4,

Fiber 3,

Carbs 24.79,

Protein 7

Veggie Bean Stew

Preparation time: 20 minutes

Cooking time: 7 hours

Servings: 8

Ingredients:

- ½ cup barley

- 1 cup black beans

- ¼ cup red beans

- 2 carrots

- 1 cup onion, chopped

- 1 cup tomato juice

- 2 potatoes

- 1 teaspoon salt

- 1 teaspoon ground black pepper

- 4 cups water

- 4 oz. tofu

- 1 teaspoon garlic powder

- 1 cup fresh cilantro

Directions:

1. Place barley, black beans, and red beans in the slow cooker vessel.

2. Add chopped onion, tomato juice, salt, ground black pepper, and garlic powder. After this, add water and close the slow cooker lid.

3. Cook the dish for 4 hours on HIGH.

4. Meanwhile, peel the carrots and cut them into the strips. Peel the potatoes and chop.

5. Add the carrot strips and chopped potatoes in the slow cooker after 4 hours of cooking.

6. Chop the fresh cilantro and add it in the slow cooker too.

7. Stir the mix and close the slow cooker lid. Cook the stew for 3 hours more on LOW.

8. Serve the prepared dish immediately or keep it in the fridge, not more than 3 days. Enjoy!

Nutrition:

Calories 207,

Fat 3.5,

Fiber 8,

Carbs 37.67,

Protein 8

Dinner Recipes

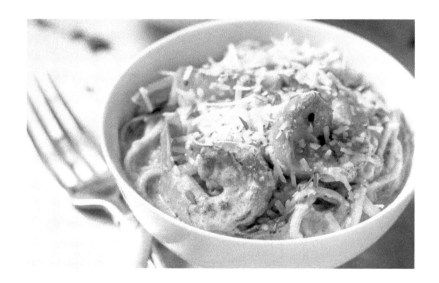

Mashed Cauliflower with Herbs

Preparation Time: 15 minutes

Cooking Time: 3-6 hours

Servings: 4

Ingredients:

- 1 cauliflower head, cut into florets
- garlic cloves, peeled
- ½ teaspoon fresh rosemary, chopped
- ½ teaspoon fresh thyme, chopped
- ½ teaspoon fresh sage, chopped
- ½ teaspoon fresh parsley, chopped
- 1 cup vegetable broth
- 2 cups water
- 1 tablespoons ghee
- Salt, pepper, to taste

Directions:

Pour broth into the slow cooker, add cauliflower florets.

Add water, it should cover the cauliflower.

Close the lid and cook on Low for 6 hours or on High for 3 hours.

Once cooked, drain water from the slow cooker.

Add herbs, salt, pepper, and ghee, puree with a blender.

Nutrition:

Calories 115

Fats 12g

Net carbs 4.7g

Protein 6.2g

Kale Quiche

Preparation Time: 15 minutes

Cooking Time: 3-5 hours

Servings: 3

Ingredients:

- 1 cup almond milk
- 4 eggs
- 1 cup Carbquick Baking Mix
- 2 cups spinach, chopped
- ½ bell pepper, chopped
- cups fresh baby kale, chopped
- 1 teaspoon garlic, chopped
- 1/3 cup fresh basil, chopped
- salt, pepper, to taste
- 1 tablespoon olive oil

Directions:

Add oil to a slow cooker or use a cooking spray.

Beat eggs into a slow cooker; add almond milk and Baking Mix, mix to combine.

Add spinach, bell pepper, garlic, and basil, stir to combine.

Close the lid and cook on Low for 5 hours or on High for 3 hours.

Make sure the quiche is done, check the center with a toothpick, it should be dry.

Nutrition :

Calories 273

Fats 24.4g

Net carbs 5.8g

Protein 10.5g

Main

Balsamic Beef

Preparation time: 20 minutes

Cooking time: 7 hours

Servings: 4

Ingredients:

- 2 tablespoons balsamic vinegar

- 1 tablespoon olive oil

- 1-pound beef loin

- 1 teaspoon minced garlic

- ½ teaspoon ground coriander

- 1 teaspoon cumin

- ½ teaspoon dried dill

- 2 tablespoons water

Directions:

Chop the beef loin roughly and place it in a large bowl, then sprinkle it with the balsamic vinegar.

Add olive oil, minced garlic, ground coriander, cumin, and dried dill.

Stir the meat well and let sit for 10 minutes.

Place the meat in the slow cooker and add water.

Close the lid and cook the beef for 7 hours on Low.

When the beef is tender, it is cooked!

Enjoy!

Nutrition:

calories 241,

fat 13.1,

fiber 0.1,

carbs 0.6,

protein 30.5

Onion Beef

Preparation time: 10 minutes

Cooking time: 5.5 hours

Servings: 14

Ingredients:

- 4-pounds beef sirloin, sliced
- 2 cups white onion, chopped
- 2 cups of water
- ½ cup butter
- 1 teaspoon ground black pepper
- 1 teaspoon salt
- 1 bay leaf

Directions

Mix beef sirloin with salt and ground black pepper and transfer to the slow cooker.

Add butter, water, onion, and bay leaf.

Close the lid and cook the meat on High for 5.5 hours.

Nutrition : 306 calories, 39.6g protein, 1.7g carbohydrates, 14.7g fat, 0.4g fiber, 133mg cholesterol, 301mg sodium, 551mg potassium.

Rosemary Leg of Lamb

Preparation time: 15 minutes Cooking time: 7 hours Servings: 8

Ingredients:

- 2-pound leg of lamb
- 1 onion
- 2 cups water
- 1 garlic clove, peeled
- 1 tablespoon mustard seeds
- 1 teaspoon salt
- ½ teaspoon turmeric
- 1 teaspoon ground black pepper

Directions:

Chop the garlic clove and combine it with the mustard seeds, turmeric, black pepper, and salt.

Peel the onion and grate it.

Mix the grated onion and spice mixture. Rub the leg of lamb with the grated onion mixture. Put the leg of lamb in the slow cooker and cook it for 7 hours on Low. Serve the cooked meal!

Nutrition: calories 225, fat 8.7, fiber 0.6, carbs 2.2, protein 32.4

Creamy Chicken Thighs

Preparation time: 15 minutes

Cooking time: 6 hours

Servings: 4

Ingredients:

* 1-pound chicken thighs, skinless

* ¼ cup almond milk, unsweetened

* 1 tablespoon full-fat cream cheese

* 1 teaspoon salt

* 1 onion, diced

* 1 teaspoon paprika

Directions:

Mix the almond milk and full-fat cream.

Add salt, diced onion, and paprika.

Stir the mixture well.

Place the chicken thighs in the slow cooker.

Add the almond milk mixture and stir it gently.

Close the slow cooker lid and cook the chicken thighs for 6 hours on High.

Transfer the cooked chicken thighs into the serving bowls and serve immediately!

Nutrition:

calories 224,

fat 14.3,

fiber 1.1,

carbs 4.7,

protein 18.9

Potato Salad

Preparation time: 10 minutes

Cooking time: 3 hours

Servings: 2

Ingredients:

- 1 cup potato, chopped
- 1 cup of water
- 1 teaspoon salt
- oz. celery stalk, chopped
- oz. fresh parsley, chopped
- ¼ onion, diced
- 1 tablespoon mayonnaise

Directions

Put the potatoes in the slow cooker. Add water and salt. Cook the potatoes on High for 3 hours. Then drain water and transfer the potatoes in the salad bowl. Add all remaining ingredients and carefully mix the salad.

Nutrition 129 calories, 5.5g protein, 12.4g carbohydrates, 6.7g fat, 2.5g fiber, 12mg cholesterol, 1479mg sodium, 465mg potassium.

Sautéed Greens

Preparation time: 15 minutes

Cooking time: 1 hour

Servings: 4

Ingredients:

- 1 cup spinach, chopped
- 2 cups collard greens, chopped
- 1 cup Swiss chard, chopped
- water
- ½ cup half and half

Directions

Put spinach, collard greens, and Swiss chard in the slow cooker.

Add water and close the lid.

Cook the greens on High for 1 hour.

Then drain water and transfer the greens in the bowl.

Bring the half and half to boil and pour over greens.

Carefully mix the greens.

Nutrition 49 calories, 1.8g protein, 3.2g carbohydrates, 3.7g fat, 1.1g fiber, 11mg cholesterol, 45mg sodium, 117mg potassium.

Soups, Stews, and Chilis

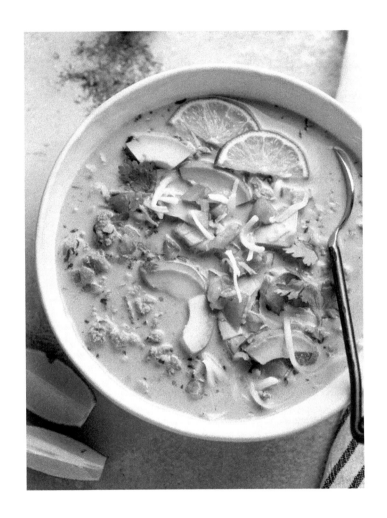

Serrano Pepper and Black Bean Soup

Preparation Time: 10 minutes

Cooking time: 10 Hours 15 Minutes Servings: 6

Ingredients:

- 2 cups dried black beans, cleaned, soaked overnight, and drained
- 4 cups organic vegetable broth
- 2 onions, chopped
- 1 cup water
- 1 tbsp. ground cumin
- 3 bay leaves
- 1 serrano pepper, finely chopped
- 2 tbsp. fresh lime juice
- 1 tsp. salt
- 1/4 cup chopped fresh cilantro
- 3 tbsp. reduced-fat sour cream

Directions:

1. Combine the beans, broth, onions, water, cumin, bay leaves, and serrano pepper in the slow cooker.

2. Cover and cook for 10 hours on LOW.

3.   Remove the bay leaves, season with salt, and stir in lime juice.

4.   Serve topped with sour cream and cilantro. Enjoy!

Nutrition: calories 286, fat 2, carbs 23, protein 17

Sweet Potato Soup

Preparation Time: 17 minutes

Cooking time: 3 hours 10 minutes

Servings: 4

Ingredients:

- 2 sweet potatoes, peeled and diced

- 1/2 onion, minced

- Garlic

- Basil

- Salt and pepper

Directions:

Place all the ingredients in a slow cooker and stir. Cover and cook for 3 hours on HIGH. Puree with an immersion blender until the soup is smooth. Serve and enjoy!

Nutrition: calories 127, fat 5, carbs 1, protein 20

Spinach Noodle Casserole

Preparation Time: 15 minutes   Cooking time: 2 hours

Servings: 5

Ingredients:

- 8 ounces dry spinach noodles
- 2 tablespoons vegetable oil
- 1 1/2 cups sour cream
- 1/3 cup all-purpose flour
- 1 1/2 cups cottage cheese
- 4 green onions, minced
- 2 teaspoons Worcestershire sauce
- 1 dash hot pepper sauce
- 2 teaspoons garlic salt

Directions:

1. In a large pot, cook noodles in the salted boiling water until they are barely tender. Drain, then rinse under the cold water. Toss with the vegetable oil.

2. In a large bowl, combine flour and sour cream while the noodles are cooking. Mix well. Stir in garlic salt, hot pepper sauce, Worcestershire sauce, green onions, and cottage cheese.

Stir the noodles into the mixture. Grease inside of the slow cooker generously. Pour in the noodle mixture. Cook, covered, for 90-120 mins on high. Nutrition: calories 226, fat 14, carbs 14, protein 8

Tasty Spiced Chili Beef Eye Roast

Preparation Time: 15 minutes

Cooking time: 8 hours

Servings: 4

Ingredients:

- 3 pounds of lean ground beef eye roast
- 2 tablespoons of Worcestershire sauce
- 4 tablespoons of fresh lime juice
- 1 ½ cups of diced onions
- 1 cup of diced red bell pepper
- 3 cloves of minced garlic
- 3 minced and seeded Serrano chilies
- Salt and pepper
- ½ cup of beef broth
- 1 cup of canned tomatoes, diced
- ½ teaspoon of dried oregano

Directions:

1. Use salt and pepper to season the beef and put it into the slow cooker. In a large bowl, whisk the remaining

ingredients together and pour them over the beef. Cook on low for 8 hours.

2.   Use 2 forks to shred the beef.

Nutrition: calories 247, fat 6, carbs 13, protein 21

Fish and Seafood

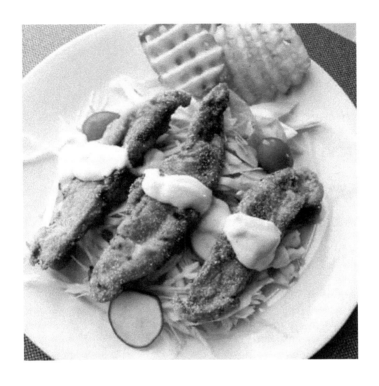

Shrimp and Salmon Skewers

Preparation Time: 10 minutes

Cooking time: 2 hours

Servings: 4

Ingredients:

- 9 oz shrimps, peeled
- 9 ounces salmon fillets, boneless and cubed
- 1 teaspoon garlic powder
- 1 teaspoon ginger powder
- 1 tablespoon lime juice
- 1/3 teaspoon oregano, dried
- 1 tablespoon sesame oil
- 1 teaspoon heavy cream
- ¾ cup of water

Directions:

1. String the shrimps and salmon into the skewers one-by-one.

2. After this, pour water into the slow cooker.

3. Arrange the shrimp and salmon skewers in the slow cooker, and add the rest of the ingredients as well.

4. Close the lid and cook shrimps for 1.5 hours on High.

5. Then transfer the cooked shrimp skewers to the plates and sprinkle with slow cooker gravy.

Nutrition: calories 185, fat 5, carbs 5, protein 14

Shrimp Salad

Preparation Time: 10 minutes

Cooking time: 30 minutes

Servings: 4

Ingredients:

- ¼ cup cherry tomatoes

- 1 cup kale, chopped

- ½ cup avocado, peeled, pitted, and cubed

- 7 oz shrimps, peeled and deveined

- 1 teaspoon basil, dried

- 3 tablespoons butter

- 1 tablespoon olive oil

- 1 tablespoon fresh parsley, chopped

- ¾ cup heavy cream

- 1 teaspoon ground black pepper

- ½ teaspoon salt

Directions:

1.   In the slow cooker, mix the shrimp with tomatoes and the other ingredients, close the lid and cook for 30 minutes on High.

2.   Divide into bowls and serve.

Nutrition: calories 248, fat 11, carbs 2, protein 8

Shrimp and Fennel Soup

Preparation Time: 10 minutes

Cooking time: 2 hours

Servings: 6

Ingredients:

- ½ cup fennel, shredded
- 12 oz shrimps, peeled
- ½ teaspoon sweet paprika
- 1 teaspoon turmeric powder
- ½ teaspoon salt
- ½ teaspoon cayenne pepper
- 1 teaspoon coriander seeds
- 2 cups of water
- 2 cups of coconut milk
- 1 teaspoon chili powder
- 1 cup spinach, chopped

Directions:

1.   In the slow cooker, mix the shrimp with fennel and the other ingredients and toss.

2.   Divide into bowls and serve.

Nutrition: calories 276, fat 6, carbs 5, protein 16

Vegetable

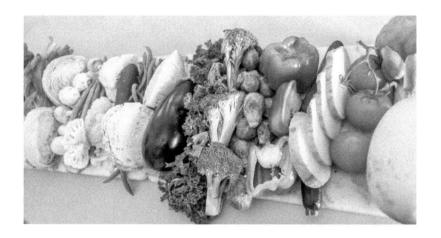

Creamy Portobello Mix

Preparation time: 15 minutes

Cooking time: 7 hours

Servings: 4

Ingredients

• 4 Portobello mushrooms

• ½ cup Monterey Jack cheese, grated

• ½ cup heavy cream

• 1 teaspoon curry powder

• 1 teaspoon basil, dried

• ½ teaspoon salt

• 1 teaspoon olive oil

Directions:

1. In the slow cooker, mix the mushrooms with the cheese and the other Ingredients.

2. Close the lid and cook the meal for 7 hours on Low.

Nutrition: calories 126, fat 5.1, fiber 1.6, carbs 5.9, protein 4.4

Eggplant Mash

Preparation time: 10 minutes

Cooking time: 2.5 hours

Servings: 2

Ingredients

- 7 oz. eggplant, trimmed

- 1 tablespoon butter

- 1 teaspoon basil, dried

- 1 teaspoon chili powder

- ½ teaspoon garlic powder

- 1/3 cup water

- ½ teaspoon salt

Directions:

1. Peel the eggplant and rub with salt.

2. Then put it in the slow cooker and water.

3. Close the lid and cook the eggplant for 2.5 hours on High.

4. Then drain water and mash the eggplant.

5. Add the rest of the Ingredients, whisk and serve.

Nutrition: calories 206, fat 6.2, fiber 3.6, carbs 7.9, protein 8.6

Cheddar Artichoke

Preparation time: 15 minutes

Cooking time: 3 hours

Servings: 6

Ingredients

- 1 teaspoon garlic, diced
- 1 tablespoon olive oil
- 1-pound artichoke hearts, chopped
- 3 oz. Cheddar cheese, shredded
- 1 teaspoon curry powder
- 1 cup chicken stock
- 1 teaspoon butter
- 1 teaspoon garam masala

Directions:

1. In the slow cooker, mix the artichokes with garlic, oil and the other Ingredients.

2. Cook the artichoke hearts for 3 hours on High.

3. Divide between plates and serve.

Nutrition: calories 135, fat 3.9, fiber 4.3, carbs 4.9, protein 4.3

Squash and Zucchinis

Preparation time: 15 minutes

Cooking time: 4 hours

Servings: 6

Ingredients

- 4 cups spaghetti squash, cubed

- 2 zucchinis, cubed

- ½ cup coconut milk

- ½ teaspoon ground cinnamon

- ¾ teaspoon ground ginger

- 3 tablespoons oregano

- 1 teaspoon butter

Directions:

1. In the slow cooker, mix the squash with the zucchinis, milk and the other Ingredients.

2. Close the lid and cook the vegetables on Low for 4 hours.

Nutrition: calories 40, fat 2.2, fiber 1.8, carbs 4.3, protein 1.1

Dill Leeks

Preparation time: 10 minutes

Cooking time: 3 hours

Servings: 3

Ingredients

- 2 cups leeks, sliced

- 1 cup chicken stock

- 2 tablespoons fresh dill, chopped

- ½ teaspoon turmeric powder

- 1 teaspoon sweet paprika

- 1 tablespoon coconut cream

- 1 teaspoon butter

Directions:

1. In the slow cooker, mix the beets with the stock, dill and the other Ingredients.

2. Cook on Low for 3 hours and serve.

Nutrition: calories 123, fat 2.9, fiber 2.2, carbs 7.5, protein 4.3.

Vegetable Lasagna

Preparation time: 20 minutes

Cooking time: 6 hours

Servings: 4

Ingredients

- 1 eggplant, sliced

- 1 cup kale, chopped

- 3 eggs, beaten

- 2 tablespoons Keto tomato sauce

- ½ teaspoon ground black pepper

- 1 cup Cheddar, grated

- ½ teaspoon chili flakes

- 1 tablespoon tomato sauce

- 1 teaspoon coconut oil

- ½ teaspoon butter

Directions:

1. Place coconut oil in the skillet and melt it.

2. Then add sliced eggplants and roast them for 1 minute from each side.

3. After this, transfer them in the bowl.

4.   Toss butter in the skillet.

5.   Place 1 beaten egg in the skillet and stir it to get the shape of a pancake.

6.   Roast the egg pancake for 1 minute from each side.

7.   Repeat the steps with remaining eggs.

8.   Separate the eggplants into 2 parts.

9.   Place 1 part of eggplants in the slow cooker. You should make the eggplant layer.

10.   Then add ½ cup chopped parsley and 1 egg pancake.

11.   Sprinkle the egg pancakes with 1/3 cup of Parmesan.

12.   Then add remaining eggplants and second egg pancake.

13.   Sprinkle it with ½ part of remaining Parmesan and top with the last egg pancake.

14.   Then spread it with tomato sauce, kale and sprinkle with chili flakes and ground black pepper.

15.   Add tomato sauce and top lasagna with remaining cheese.

16.   Close the lid and cook lasagna for 6 hours on Low.

Nutrition: calories 257, fat 15.9, fiber 4.5, carbs 10.5, protein 21.5

Meat

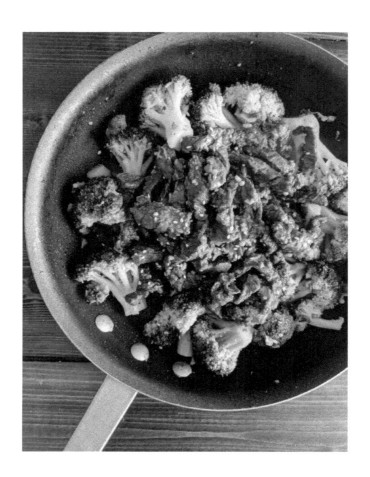

Beef and Artichokes Bowls

Preparation time: 10 minutes

Cooking time: 7 hours

Servings: 2

Ingredients

- oz. beef sirloin, chopped
- ½ teaspoon cayenne pepper
- ½ teaspoon white pepper
- artichoke hearts, chopped
- 1 cup of water
- 1 teaspoon salt

Directions

1   Mix meat with white pepper and cayenne pepper. Transfer it to the slow cooker bowl.

2   Add salt, artichoke hearts, and water.

3   Close h lid and cook the meal on Low for 7 hours.

Nutrition : 313 calories, 36.5g protein, 4.6g carbohydrates, 5.9g fat, 17.8g fiber, 76mg cholesterol, 1527mg sodium, 1559mg potassium.

Mustard Beef

Preparation time: 10 minutes Cooking time: 8 hours

Servings: 4 Ingredients

- 1-pound beef sirloin, chopped
- 1 tablespoon capers, drained
- 1 cup of water
- 2 tablespoons mustard
- 1 tablespoon coconut oil

Directions

1   Mixmeat with mustard and leave for 10 minutes to marinate.

2   Then melt the coconut oil in the skillet.

3   Add meat and roast it for 1 minute per side on high heat.

4   After this, transfer the meat to the slow cooker.

5   Add water and capers.

6   Cook the meal on Low for 8 hours.

Nutrition : 267 calories, 35.9g protein, 2.1g carbohydrates, 12.1g fat, 0.9g fiber, 101mg cholesterol, 140mg sodium, 496mg potassium.

Beef Masala

Preparation time: 15 minutes

Cooking time: 9 hours

Servings: 6

Ingredients

- 1-pound beef sirloin, sliced

- 1 teaspoon gram masala

- 2 tablespoons lemon juice

- 1 teaspoon ground paprika

- ½ cup of coconut milk

- 1 teaspoon dried mint

Directions

1   In the bowl, mix coconut milk with dried mint, ground paprika, lemon juice, and gram masala. Then add beef sirloin and mix the mixture. Leave it for at least 10 minutes to marinate.

2   Then transfer the mixture to the slow cooker. Cook it on Low for 9 hours.

Nutrition : 283 calories, 35.3g protein, 2.2g carbohydrates, 14.4g fat, 0.9g fiber, 101mg cholesterol, 82mg sodium, 560mg potassium.

Beef Sauté with Endives

Preparation time: 10 minutes Cooking time: 8 hours

Servings: 4 Ingredients

- 1-pound beef sirloin, chopped

- oz. endives, roughly chopped

- 1 teaspoon peppercorns

- 1 carrot, diced

- 1 onion, sliced

- 1 cup of water

- ½ cup tomato juice

Directions

1 Mix beef with onion, carrot, and peppercorns.

2 Place the mixture in the slow cooker. Add water and tomato juice. Then close the lid and cook it on High for 5 hours. After this, add endives and cook the meal for 3 hours on Low.

Nutrition : 238 calories, 35.4g protein, 6.4g carbohydrates, 7.2g fat, 1.9g fiber, 101mg cholesterol, 175mg sodium, 689mg potassium.

Sweet Beef

Preparation time: 10 minutes

Cooking time: 5 hours

Servings: 4

Ingredients

- 1-pound beef roast, sliced

- 1 tablespoon maple syrup

- 2 tablespoons lemon juice

- 1 teaspoon dried oregano

- 1 cup of water

Directions

1   Mix water with maple syrup, lemon juice, and dried oregano.

2   Then pour the liquid into the slow cooker.

3   Add beef roast and close the lid.

4   Cook he meal on High for 5 hours.

Nutrition : 227 calories, 34.5g protein, 3.8g carbohydrates, 7.2g fat, 0.2g fiber, 101mg cholesterol, 78mg sodium, 483mg potassium.

Thyme Beef

Preparation time: 15 minutes

Cooking time: 5 hours

Servings: 2

Ingredients

- oz. beef sirloin, chopped

- 1 tablespoon dried thyme

- 1 tablespoon olive oil

- ½ cup of water

- 1 teaspoon salt

Directions

1   Preheat the skillet well. Then mix beef with dried thyme and olive oil.

2   Put the meat in the hot skillet and roast for 2 minutes per side on high heat.

3   Then transfer the meat to the slow cooker.

4   Add salt and water. Cook the meal on High for 5 hours.

Nutrition : 274 calories, 34.5g protein 0.9g carbohydrates, 14.2g fat, 0.5g fiber 101mg cholesterol, 1240mg sodium, 469mg potassium

Side Dish Recipes

Garlic Butter Green Beans

Preparation time: 15 minutes

Cooking time: 2 Hours

Servings: 6

Ingredients

- 22 ounces green beans

- 2 garlic cloves, minced

- ¼ cup butter, soft

- 2 tablespoons parmesan, grated

Directions:

1. In your Crock Pot, mix green beans with garlic, butter and parmesan, toss, cover and cook on High for 2 hours.

2. Divide between plates, sprinkle parmesan all over and serve as a side dish.

Nutrition: calories 60, fat 4, fiber 1, carbs 3, protein 1

Green Beans and Red Peppers

Preparation time: 15 minutes

Cooking time: 2 Hours

Servings: 2

Ingredients

- 2 cups green beans, halved
- 1 red bell pepper, cut into strips
- Salt and black pepper to the taste
- 1 tablespoon olive oil
- 1 and ½ tablespoon honey mustard

Directions:

1. In your Crock Pot, mix green beans with bell pepper, salt, pepper, oil and honey mustard, toss, cover and cook on High for 2 hours.

2. Divide between plates and serve as a side dish.

Nutrition: calories 50, fat 0, fiber 4, carbs 8, protein 2

Cauliflower Carrot Gratin

Preparation time: 15 minutes

Cooking time: 7 Hours

Servings: 12

Ingredients

- 16 oz. baby carrots
- 6 tbsp. butter, soft
- 1 cauliflower head, florets separated
- Salt and black pepper to the taste
- 1 yellow onion, chopped
- 1 tsp. mustard powder
- 1 and ½ cups of milk
- 6 oz. cheddar cheese, grated
- ½ cup breadcrumbs

Directions:

1. Add carrots, cauliflower, and rest of the Ingredients: to the Crock Pot.

2. Put the cooker's lid on and set the cooking time to 7 hours on Low settings.

3. Serve warm.

Nutrition: Per Serving: Calories: 182, Total Fat: 4g, Fiber: 7g, Total Carbs: 9g, Protein: 4g

Minty Peas and Tomatoes

Preparation time: 15 minutes

Cooking time: 3 Hours

Servings: 2

Ingredients

- 1 pound okra, sliced
- ½ pound tomatoes, cut into wedges
- 1 tablespoon olive oil
- ½ cup veggie stock
- ½ teaspoon chili powder
- Salt and black pepper to the taste
- 1 tablespoon mint, chopped
- 3 green onions, chopped
- 1 tablespoon chives, chopped

Directions:

1.   Grease your Crock Pot with the oil, and mix the okra with the tomatoes and the other Ingredients: inside.

2.   Put the lid on, cook on Low for 3 hours, divide between plates and serve as a side dish.

Nutrition: calories 70, fat 1, fiber 1, carbs 4, protein 6

Lemon Artichokes

Preparation time: 15 minutes

Cooking time: 3 Hours

Servings: 2

Ingredients

*   1 cup veggie stock

*   2 medium artichokes, trimmed

*   1 tablespoon lemon juice

*   1 tablespoon lemon zest, grated

*   Salt to the taste

Directions:

1.   In your Crock Pot, mix the artichokes with the stock and the other Ingredients, and then toss it, put the lid on and cook on Low for 3 hours.

2.   Divide artichokes between plates and serve as a side dish.

Nutrition: calories 100, fat 2, fiber 5, carbs 10, protein 4

Mashed Potatoes

Preparation time: 15 minutes

Cooking time: 6 Hours

Servings: 2

Ingredients

- 1 pound gold potatoes, peeled and cubed
- 2 garlic cloves, chopped
- 1 cup milk
- 1 cup water
- 2 tablespoons butter
- A pinch of salt and white pepper

Directions:

1.   In your Crock Pot, mix the potatoes with the water, salt and pepper, put the lid on and cook on Low for 6 hours.

2.   Mash the potatoes; add the rest of the Ingredients, whisk and serve.

Nutrition: calories 135, fat 4, fiber 2, carbs 10, protein 4

Appetizers & Snacks

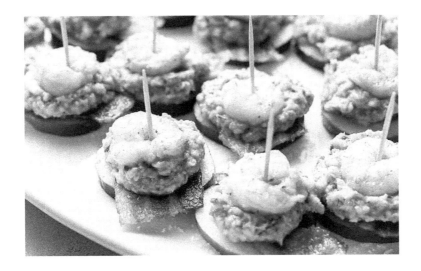

Buffalo Chicken Meatballs

Preparation time: 15 minutes

Cooking time: 2 hours & 5 minutes

Servings: 4

Ingredients

- 1-pound ground grass-fed chicken

- 1 organic egg

- 1/3 cup almond meal

- scallions, sliced thinly

- 2 garlic cloves, minced

- Salt

- black pepper, ground

- ¾ cup sugar-free buffalo sauce

Directions:

1   Preheat the oven to 400 degrees F.

2   In a bowl, add all Ingredients except buffalo sauce and mix until well combined.

3   Make 1½-inch balls from chicken mixture.

4   Arrange meatballs onto a baking sheet and bake for about 5 minutes.

5   Remove from oven and transfer meatballs into a slow cooker with buffalo sauce, stir.

6   Cook on low, then covered, for about 2 hours. Serve immediately.

Nutrition:

Calories: 283

Carbohydrates: 3g

Protein: 36.1g

Fat: 13.5g

Sugar: 0.6g

Sodium: 224mg

Fiber: 1.2g

Foolproof Beef Meatballs

Preparation time: 15 minutes

Cooking time: 7 hours & 5 minutesServings: 8

Ingredients

- pounds ground lean grass-fed beef

- 2 organic eggs, beaten

- 1 medium yellow onion, chopped

- 2 garlic cloves, minced

- ¼ cup fresh parsley leaves, chopped

- ½ teaspoon red pepper flakes, crushed

- ¼ teaspoon cayenne pepper

- Salt

- ground black pepper

- 2 tablespoons olive oil

Directions:

1   Mix items except oil in a bowl. Make desired size balls from the mixture.

2   Heat-up oil over medium-high heat in a large skillet, then cook meatballs for 4-5 minutes or until golden brown from all sides.

3   Transfer the meatballs into a greased slow cooker.

4   Cook in the slow cooker on low, covered, for about 7 hours. Serve hot.

Nutrition:

Calories: 264

Carbohydrates: 10.8g

Protein: 36.1g

Fat: 11.7g

Sugar: 0.7g

Sodium: 508mg

Fiber: 0g

Super-Tasty Pork Meatballs

Preparation time: 15 minutes

Cooking time: 6 hours & 20 minutes

Servings: 8

Ingredients

- pounds lean ground pork
- 1 cup Cheddar cheese, shredded
- 1 large organic egg
- ¼ cup yellow onion, chopped
- ¼ teaspoon ground allspice
- 1 tablespoon water
- tablespoons unsalted butter
- 1½ cups heavy whipping cream
- 1½ cups homemade chicken broth
- 1 tablespoon Worcestershire sauce
- 1 tablespoon Dijon mustard

Directions:

1   Warm-up, the oven to 400 degrees F, then line a large baking dish with parchment paper.

2   In a large bowl, add ground pork, cheddar cheese, egg, onion, allspice, and water and mix until well combined.

3   Make 1½-inch balls from pork mixture.

4   Arrange the meatballs onto a prepared baking dish and bake for about 20 minutes.

5   Meanwhile, in a small skillet, add butter, heavy cream, and broth and bring to a gentle boil over medium heat.

6   Adjust to low and simmer for about 20 minutes, stirring occasionally.

7   Stir in Worcestershire sauce and mustard and remove from heat.

8   In a slow cooker, add sauce and meatballs and stir.

9   Cook in the slow cooker on low, covered, for about 4-6 hours. Serve immediately.

Nutrition: Calories: 358Carbohydrates: 1.9gProtein: 29.2gFat: 25.8gSugar: 0.8gSodium: 398mgFiber: 0.2g

Inspiring Sausage Sliders

Preparation time: 15 minutesCooking time: 5 hoursServings: 10

Ingredients

- cups sugar-free ketchup

- ¼ cup Erythritol

- 1 tablespoon Worcestershire sauce

- 2 teaspoons mustard

- 1 teaspoon hot sauce

- 1 medium yellow onion, chopped finely

- ½ cup homemade chicken broth

- 2 pounds pork sausage, cut into ½-inch rounds

Directions:

1 In a large slow cooker, add all items and stir to combine. Cook on low, covered, for about 4-5 hours. Serve immediately.

Nutrition:Calories: 365Carbohydrates: 13.7gProtein: 19gFat: 26.2gSugar: 11.8gSodium: 1280mgFiber: 0.5g

Potluck Party Peppers

Preparation time: 15 minutesCooking time: 9 hours

Servings: 10

Ingredients

- 1½ pounds mini sweet peppers, seeded and tops removed
- 1-pound ground Italian sausage
- 1 (24-ounce) jar sugar-free spaghetti sauce
- 8-ounce mozzarella cheese, shredded

Directions:

1	Stuff each pepper evenly with sausage.

2	Lightly greased slow cooker, arrange peppers. Cook on low, covered, for about 6-8 hours.

3	Uncover the slow cooker and top each pepper with mozzarella cheese.

4	Cook, covered for about 10 minutes. Serve hot.

Nutrition:Calories: 248Carbohydrates: 9.6gProtein: 15.6gFat: 16gSugar: 7.5gSodium: 824mgFiber: 1.8g

Perfect Eggplant Tapenade

Preparation time: 15 minutesCooking time: 9 hours

Servings: 2 Ingredients

- cups eggplants, chopped

- 1 cup tomatoes, chopped

- garlic cloves, minced

- 2 teaspoons capers

- 2 teaspoons fresh lemon juice

- 1 teaspoon dried basil

- Salt, to taste

- Pinch of ground black pepper

Directions:In a slow cooker, add eggplant, tomatoes, garlic, and capers and mix well. Cook on low, covered, for about 7-9 hours. Uncover the slow cooker and stir in the remaining IngredientsServe hot.

Nutrition:Calories: 46Carbohydrates: 10.1g Protein: 2g Fat: 0.4g Sugar: 5g Sodium: 170mg Fiber: 4.2g

Desserts

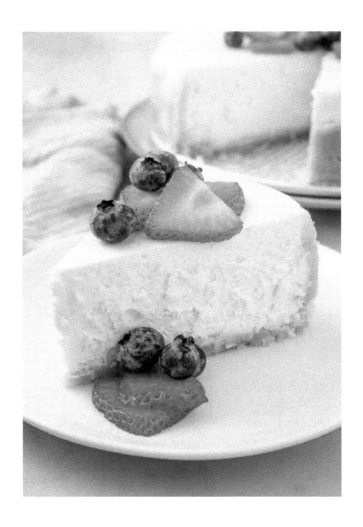

Delicious Chocolate Peanut Butter Fudge

Preparation Time: 17 minutes

Cooking time: 2 hours

Servings: 12

Ingredients:

- Coconut oil, for coating the slow cooker insert

- 1½ cups heavy (whipping) cream

- 1 cup all-natural peanut butter

- 1 tablespoon unsalted butter, melted

- 1 teaspoon pure vanilla extract

- 4 ounces unsweetened chocolate, chopped

- ½ cup erythritol

- 1 teaspoon stevia powder

Directions:

1. Generously coat the inside of the slow cooker insert with coconut oil.

2. In the slow cooker, stir together the heavy cream, peanut butter, butter, vanilla, chocolate, erythritol, and stevia. Cover and cook for 2 hours on low, stirring occasionally.

3.   Line a small, rimmed baking sheet with parchment or wax paper.

4.   Transfer the cooked fudge to the prepared sheet and refrigerate it for at least 4 hours.

5.   Cut into squares and serve chilled.

Nutrition: calories 246, fat 23, carbs 7, protein 9

Lightning Source UK Ltd.
Milton Keynes UK
UKHW022050220321
380813UK00004B/603